Free from Fat

Discover easy answers
to good health with
low fat eating and a
strength training program

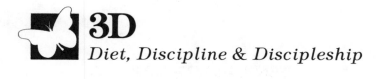

3D
Diet, Discipline & Discipleship

1st Printing,   August 1993
2nd Printing,   November 1993

ISBN #: 1-55725-030-8
Library of Congress Card Catalog No.: 93-60945

Table of Contents

Introduction

Ready for some good news?

Are you tired of thinking negatively about yourself? Is most of your negativity centered about who you are, and what you weigh? Have you been on more diets than you can count on both hands? Are you literally "dieted" to death and very discouraged about the long-lasting results? If you answered yes to all of the above, chances are, on top of all of those feelings, you're frustrated that the older you get, the harder it is to get the weight off!

Believe me, we understand! Diet, Discipline and Discipleship (3D) is now 21 years old, and more than 300,000 people have been through the program. There are groups on the coast of Maine, the top of Alaska, in Portugal, Spain and South America, throughout the U.K. and all the way down in Australia! In all of those groups, people like you have counted on 3D to be more than just another diet program, and their testimonies have confirmed that it is indeed. Participants have gained inner healing, found a tremendous support group, and learned how to pray with others. . . forgive themselves . . . and keep pressing on with God. Best of all, they have discovered how faithfully He meets the needs of all who sincerely turn to Him. (And literally tons of weight have been lost in the process!)

5

But—for all that success, a lot of us old-timers need something fresh *now*, to pick up the pace and recharge our batteries. Well, it's here! A breakthrough in health perception—and once again, 3D is on the cutting edge!

Our new dimension is the latest and very best solution that the medical profession, researchers and health scientists have come up with, in answer to questions about diet, aging, health and weight—a low-fat food intake program, combined with resistance-training exercise. Each of these concepts has been making headlines recently, and together they are an absolute winner! While there is nothing magical about the combination, we are already finding dramatic results in our pilot groups—and we can say with assurance that it will revitalize and refresh you, and challenge you with new answers for old problems. For example, it banishes the dismal image of dieting and restores the original meaning of the word, diet: "daily food intake." So buckle up and let's resist the temptation to rebel against "dieting." Why become a member of the anti-diet movement? Why remain guilty, depressed and negative about ourselves? Apply 3D's new answers—to keep us moving in God's direction of bringing *all* aspects of our lives under the Lordship of Christ.

In these pages, you'll learn about fats—exactly what they are and how to limit your daily intake of them. You'll also learn a new and exciting exercise program that will change your whole attitude about exercise. In this program, you will count fats instead of food exchanges or calories. You'll keep a daily diary of the number of fats found in your breakfast, lunch and dinner, and, of course, in your snacks. And as for strength training, believe it or not, you will be lifting weights, as well as doing aerobic exercises! The bottom line is your body will get a new message: Go after **stored** fat for energy.

Warning: There is nothing easy or superficial about this new plan. But there *is* something very promising and exciting about it—as you will experience, as soon as you get into it.

This supplementary guide will provide you with information on fats as well as instructions in resistance training exercise. We do want to remind you, however, that the meat of the 3D program is the daily devotional workbook and your commitment to prayer and Bible reading. Written with an understanding of practical problems and a challenge to spiritual growth, these ingredients are essential to a balanced approach to meet our needs, whether they be as practical as losing some weight or as serious as family problems.

You are about to change some habit patterns and this takes time and perseverance.

You have our support as an organization, our prayers as fellow sojourners, and our promise that this will be the most challenging and exciting adventure you have embarked on in the health department of your life.

You can expect to feel better, look better and know beyond a shadow of a doubt that your body is on its way to being fit for His kingdom as never before!

From the beginning 3D has been built around the very best food plan there is—the exchange diet developed by the American Diabetic & Dietetic Association. Highly recommended by doctors and dieticians, the concept of regulating daily food intake by the "basic four" groups rather than by calorie content was introduced in the early 1950's. The exchange groups—meats, vegetables and fruits, dairy and grains—were to be a basic part of each meal, with portions proposed for each category. Considered a "healthy diet plan," it was altered as necessary for people with particular health problems. Within the 3D program, people made a commitment to this balanced "diet" plan and did indeed lose weight gradually and realistically.

But science was marching on during those twenty years; medical researchers all over the world were discovering new facts regarding diet and health. For the medical profession was facing a critical situation: more Americans were dying of heart attacks and heart disease than ever before. The best-fed country in the whole world was in a health crisis! Why?

It was obvious that everyone, experts as well as laymen, had a lot more to learn about diet—daily food intake. So we began to search for fresh insights that could be added to the 3D program. We studied the publications from The American Heart Foundation, the National Dairy Association, and the Department of Agriculture. We scanned medical articles and nutritional newsletters coming out of universities and medical schools. We visited the USDA Human Nutrition Research Center on Aging at Tufts University.

We even decided to form some experimental groups with seasoned 3D members and implement the new insights we were gathering into the 3D format. Needless to say, a few of us were hoping the new information would fix us up fast, especially in the weight control department.

Would this new fat-free dieting be the answer we were all secretly looking for to put an end to the seemingly endless struggle? Yes, as far as we are concerned, it is the missing ingredient to keeping weight off! So let's start by looking at some "fat facts."

A New Challenge: Counting Grams of Fat

What is fat?

"Fat" is, unfortunately, essential. It is necessary to the health of people of all ages, a principal source of energy which carries vitamins A, D, E and K. The amount of fat an adult requires, however, is low and easily fulfilled with a well-rounded diet. Most of us eat far more fat than necessary.

Fats and carbohydrates are made up of the same elements— carbon, hydrogen and oxygen, but fats being a more concentrated form of fuel, contain more carbon and less oxygen than carbohydrates. For this reason, a gram of fat supplies 9 calories, where a gram of carbohydrates supplies 4. You will gain more weight eating fat, than you would eating the same amount of carbohydrates.

Another interesting difference between these fuels, is how the body stores them. Carbohydrates are transformed into glycogen, and stored in a solution of water—4 parts water to 1 part glycogen. So, when you decrease your carbohydrate intake, you will lose weight, but it is mostly water you are losing—a fact on which weight loss diets are based. The moment you increase your carbohydrate intake at all, however, you will gain back the weight as quickly as you lost it.

9

Another reason carbohydrates are quickly lost is that there is very little space in the body set apart for storing carbohydrates—and there are vast storage areas for fats. What's more, the body stores this fat in a very concentrated way—in fact, the ratio of fat to water is reversed: 4 parts fat to 1 part water. So the weight you lose when you cut down on fats is real weight loss, and not just water.

It's the fat that makes us fat. Dietary fat enters the body in a form ready-made for storage that requires no extra work or conversion. Thus, if the body takes in 10 fat calories, it may simply store those 10 fat calories as is, especially if there is already a surplus of fat in your diet, and your body has all the energy it needs. With carbohydrates it is a different story: carbohydrates calories *must* be converted to glycogen to be used by the body. This conversion process takes energy, and energy burns calories! But fat calories slide quickly and easily into our fat cells with no extra work or difficulty. You eat 10, you keep 10.

Our bodies regard fat as a source for energy, and can come from two sources: from our diet, or from our existing fat cells. If you eat a high-fat diet, you will get the energy you need, but any excess fat will just go into your cells and make you fat. What happens if you cut down on your fat intake? After your body has used up the available glycogen, it will meet its energy needs by drawing on its reserves of stored fat. Given a choice, your body prefers to get its energy from the fat in your diet, than from the carbohydrates; but, if you cut back on fats, and make sure you are getting regular, aerobic exercise, eventually your body is going to be forced to use fat that it has already stored.

Now we need to learn how to find these fats in our diet, and to do that, let's take a look at the food groups.

Fats in the Basic Four Food Groups

Here is where you can find fat—and some hints on what to avoid.

Dairy Products   60-90% fat

Unfortunately most dairy products are almost entirely fat, and this includes eggs, yogurt, cheese, butter, milk, diet margarine and vegetable oil. For dairy products the best bet is to use low-fat or no-fat items like "egg beaters" in recipes instead of eggs, or for frying, to use non-stick sprays instead of butter or margarine.

Meat   10-80% fat

Beef and lamb run 50-80% fat. And unfortunately, just trimming the fat off beef or lamb will not make much difference as the fat is throughout the meat. But turkey and chicken (with the skin off) is a good alternate choice usually only 20-40% fat. And keep in mind that light meat is lower in fat than dark meat. Finally what is the best choice and the worst? Pork is the worst choice: 80% fat. But fish is excellent: usually no more than 10-20% fat.

Grains   10-20% fat

Most grains, cereals, and pasta are less than 20% fat, and, in general, breads are 10-20% fat. Cookies, cakes and muffins, however, are usually made with ingredients like butter which greatly increases the fat content. And sad to say, you'll have to stay away from nuts, seeds, and peanut butter which surprisingly are 70-90% fat.

Vegetables and Fruits   0% fat

Almost all vegetables are virtually fat free, so you can eat as many of those as you wish! A few, however, like avocado and coconut are very high in fatty oils. Some vegetables and fruits do have a gram of fat—banana, corn on the cob, pears, winter squash, but one gram of fat is not going to be a problem.

Hints on Reducing Fat

There are some very practical and simple ways to reduce the number of grams of fat you have in your daily food plan. Listed on this page are some helpful hints that will help you achieve your goal of a low fat food plan.

- Use only no-fat dairy products
- Drink skim milk only
- Frozen yogurt instead of ice cream
- Egg beaters instead of eggs
- Substitute egg whites for whole eggs in baking (2 egg whites for 1 egg)
- Jam, instead of butter on toast (sugar free jam is lower in calories, but regular jam is okay).
- Broil, or bake things instead of frying (an easy way to cut out cooking oils)
- Choose a hard roll, pita bread or whole wheat bread instead of a croissant
- Turkey, chicken or fish instead of beef
- Choose ground beef, onions, peppers and mushrooms on your pizzi instead of sausage or pepperoni
- Remove the skin from chicken and turkey
- Substitute no-fat yogurt for sour cream in baking
- Sauté vegetables in liquids—soy sauce, chicken broth
- Hot dogs instead of Polish or Italian sausage (Chicken or turkey hot dogs are even better!)
- Water-packed tuna instead of oil-packed tuna
- Eat lots of vegetables and cut down on meat intake
- Substitute cocoa with diet margarine for baking chocolate in recipes
- Try Oriental cuisine—less animal fat in cooking and high in rice and vegetables
- Don't eat nuts

- Snack on unbuttered popcorn or pretzels instead of potato chips
- Eat hard candy or mint if you have a sweet craving
- For desserts, try no-fat desserts at supermarket
- Eat lots of fruits
- Look for recipes that use applesauce and crushed pineapple in place of butter/oil

3D would like to challenge you to count grams of fats for three months. Instead of keeping a daily food sheet, keep a "fat diary" (found in the back of this guide)—recording all grams of fat eaten daily. It will be necessary to read labels carefully and refer to this guide daily, but after 3 months you will *know* the fat facts as well as you know the food exchanges. You should keep your fat intake at no more than 30% of your overall calories. If you are eating 1200 calories per day, then no more than 360 calories should be fat. Since each gram of fat is 9 calories, the grams of fat you need to _maintain_ your weight would be 40 grams. 3D recommends that women who want to lose weight during this 12-week session eat no more than 30 grams of fat and no less than 20. (Men should eat a maximum of 65 and a minimum of 50 grams of fat).

You can learn to budget fat the same way you budget money—spending on whatever foods you like but staying within your budget. There are no "good" foods or "bad" foods, but every food needs to fit into your daily fat budget. If you choose to have 1/2 cup of ice cream, you must use 10 grams of your fat allowance. You decide if it's worth it. As far as calories are concerned, fat is fat. The fat in ice cream is no worse than the fat in bacon or cheddar cheese—or, believe it or not, whole milk.

Fat Budget

Below is a fat budget plan showing you different choices. One is worked out for 30% fat calories, the second for 25%, and the third is 20%. Now here is the really hard part: you should not go any lower than the lowest figure on this chart for your daily calorie allowance. Fat *is* essential in your diet to maintain normal metabolism—too little fat is not good. After looking over the chart, pray and decide what you should do for the next 12 weeks—and fill in the sentence at the bottom of the page with your commitment.

Fat Budget Plan

Daily Caloric Allowance	1000	1200	1500	1850	2000	2400
30% Fat Calories (Daily calories $\times$ .3)	300	360	450	555	600	720
# Fat Grams allowed (Fat calories $\div$ 9)	33	40	50	62	67	80

Daily Caloric Allowance	1000	1200	1500	1850	2000	2400
25% Fat Calories (Daily calories $\times$ .25)	250	300	375	463	500	600
# Fat Grams allowed (Fat calories $\div$ 9)	28	33	41	51	55	67

Daily Caloric Allowance	1000	1200	1500	1850	2000	2400
20% Fat Calories (Daily calories $\times$ .2)	200	240	300	370	400	480
# Fat Grams allowed (Fat calories $\div$ 9)	22	26	33	41	44	53

My Personal Fat Budget should be _____ grams of fat for the first 12 weeks of 3D. It is _____% of _____ calories daily.

Now that you have a general idea of where to find the fats hidden in the four food groups, the following pages offer a wise, categorized sampling of food, together with a listing of combination foods with their grams of fat. These lists will help you quickly find specific foods and the grams of fat for each item. Also included with this guide is a color-coated chart published by the American Heart Association that you can put on your refrigerator. At a quick glance, you will be able to differentiate between higher fat foods and low fat foods.

Fats in Everyday Foods

(Please use these tables as a guide. To count specific fats in your diet, we suggest you read labels carefully.)

DAIRY PRODUCTS

No fat or trace amounts	milk—evap. skim, ½ c. yogurt—plain nonfat, 8-oz.
1-3 grams of fat	butter—whipped, 1 t. buttermilk, 1 c. cottage cheese—1%, 1 c. half & half, 1 T. milk—1%, 1 c. sour cream, 1 T. yogurt—vanilla lowfat, 8-oz.
4-6 grams of fat	butter, 1 t. cottage cheese—2%, 1 c. milk—2%, 1 c. mozarella, 1 oz. vanilla ice milk, 1 c. yogurt—plain lowfat, 8-oz.
7-10 grams of fat	yogurt—plain, 8-oz. gouda cheese, 1 oz. milk—whole, 1 c. Swiss cheese, 1 oz. American cheese, 1 oz. cheddar cheese, 1 oz. monterey Jack cheese, 1 oz. muenster cheese, 1 oz. cream cheese, 1 oz. milk—evaporated, ½ c. milk—goat, 1 c.
11+ grams of fat	custard—baked, 1 c. (17 g.) ricotta, ½ c. (16 g.) vanilla ice cream, 1 c. (16% fat-24 g.)

FRUITS/VEGETABLES (most fruits and vegetables contain no fat)

No fat or trace amounts	apple beets broccoli carrots cauliflower eggplant grapes green beans lettuce lima beans onion orange peas pineapple potato squash strawberries tomato zucchini
1 gram	banana blueberries (1 c. fresh) chickpeas, ½ c. corn, ½ c. corn on the cob (1 ear) pear
4-6 grams of fat	
7-10 grams of fat	
11+ grams of fat	avocado (14 g.) coconut—shredded, ½ c (16 g.)

GRAINS

No fat or trace amounts	brown rice, ½ c brown bread (canned) cellophane noodles corn flakes, 1 oz. cream of wheat melba toast, plain rice cakes rice krispies shredded wheat white rice, ½ c puffed wheat or rice
1-3 grams of fat	bagel barley, ¼ c. breadsticks, 1 plain cheese crackers, 10 (1/3 oz.) corn grits, 1 c. dinner roll english muffin french bread (1 slice) graham crackers (2 squares) hamburger roll hot dog roll noodles, egg, cooked, 1 c. oatmeal, cooked, 1 c. pancake, plain, 1 (4" dia.) pasta, 2 oz. pita bread, 1 (6" dia.) saltines, 4 spaghetti noodles white bread/whole wheat bread (1 slice)
4-6 grams of fat	biscuit, 1 oz. blueberry muffin, 1 bran muffin, 1 corn muffin, 1 toaster pastries, 1
7-10 grams of fat	granola, ¼ c. waffle mix w/egg & milk, 1
11+ grams of fat	chow mein noodles, 1 c. (14 g.)

MEATS

No fat or trace amounts	egg, white only
1-3 grams of fat	bacon, 1 strip baked beans (plain), ½ c. bass, 3 oz. blackeye peas, 1 c. chicken breast (½-w/o skin), 3 oz. clams, 3 oz. cod, 1 fillet corned beef, 1 slice crab-alaska king, 3 oz. haddock, 1 fillet, 5 oz. kidney beans, 1 c. lentils, 1 c. lobster, 3 oz. oysters, raw 6 med. pepperoni, 1 slice, 2 oz. perch, 3 oz. pinto beans, 1 c. pollack, 3 oz. red beans, ½ c. refried beans, 4 oz. salami-hard, 1 slice, 1/3 oz. scallops, 3 oz. shrimp, 3 oz. snapper, 3 oz. sole, 3 oz. tuna—light in water, 3 oz. tuna—white in water, 3 oz.
4-6 grams of fat	bluefish, 3 oz. chicken-light meat w/o skin, 3 oz. egg, poached egg, hard cooked halibut, ½ fillet, 5 oz. liver pate, 1 T liver-beef, 3 oz. oysters-steamed, 3 oz. salami, 1 oz. sausage-pork & beef, ½ oz. tofu-regular, ½ c.

MEATS (continued)

4-6 grams of fat	turkey-light meat w/o skin, 3 oz. veal cutlet, lean only whitefish, 3 oz.
7-10 grams of fat	beef-bottom round, trim 0", 3 oz. bologna, 1 oz. chicken livers, 1 c. ham center slice (lean only), 4 oz. ham boneless (11% fat), 3 oz. ham-canned (extra lean), 1 oz. hot dog (turkey), 1.5 oz. kielbasa, 1 oz. lamb (lean only) cubed, 3 oz. liverwurst, 1 oz. pork chop (lean only), 2.1 oz. porterhouse steak (lean only), 3 oz. trout, 3 oz. tuna—light in oil, 3 oz. tuna—white in oil, 3 oz. turkey-dark meat w/o skin, 3 oz. veal sirloin (lean only), 3 oz.
11+ grams of fat	almonds, 1 oz. (15 g.) bratwurst, pk & bf, 1 link (19 g.) brazil nuts, 1 oz. (19 g.) cashews, 1 oz. (13 g.) chicken-dark meat w/o skin, 1 c. (13 g.) chuck roast, 3 oz. (21 g.) corned beef brisket, 3 oz. (16 g.) ground beef (extra lean), 3 oz. (14 g.) ground beef (lean), 3 oz. (16 g.) ground beef (reg.), 3 oz. (18 g.) herring, 5 oz. (17 g.) hot dog-beef, 1.5 oz. (13 g.) lamb ground, 3 oz. (17 g.) lamb-roasted, 3 oz. (14 g.) macadamia nuts, 1 oz. (22 g.) mackerel, 3 oz. (15 g.) peanut butter, 2 T. (16 g.) peanuts-dry roast, 1 oz. (15 g.) peanuts-oil roast, 1 oz. (16 g.)

MEATS (continued)

11+ grams of fat	pecans-dry roast, 1 oz.(18 g.) pecans-oil roasted, 1 oz. (20 g.) pistachios-dry roasted, 1 oz. (15 g.) pork loin (lean only) 3 oz. (12 g.) pot roast-trim 0", 3 oz. (13 g.) soybeans-cooked, 1 c. (15 g.) soybeans-dry roast, ½ c.(19 g.) turkey wing w/skin, (23 g.)

OTHER

No fat or trace amounts	angel food cake catsup coffee fruit jellies/jams garlic hard candy herb teas herbs/spices honey jello marshmallow mustard olives, ripe pickles popcorn—air-popped salsa soda soy sauce sugar syrups vinegar
1-3 grams of fat	beef broth, 1 c. chicken broth, 1 c. date nut bread, ½" slice diet margarine, 1 t. non-dairy whipped topping, 1 T.

OTHER (continued)

1-3 grams of fat	nutmeg, 1 t. olives—green, 4 med. popcorn popped w/veg oil, 1 c. teriyaki sauce, 1 c. chicken noodle soup,* 1 c. clam chowder, New Eng.,* 1 c. tomato soup,* 1 c. *with water or skim milk
4-6 grams of fat	barbecue sauce, 1 c. brownie, 8 oz. margarine, 1 t. rice pudding, ½ c. salad dressing—1,000 Island, 1 T. salad dressing—French, 1 T. sandwich spread, 1 T. scalloped potatoes, ½ c sherbert, 1 c tapioca pudding, ½ c vanilla pudding, ½ c.
7-10 grams of fat	almond butter, 1 T corn chips, 1 oz. eclair, 1 hash browns, ½ c. hot cocoa, 1 c jelly doughnut, 1 oatmeal raisin cookies, 4 (1.8 oz.) pizza, 1 slice (1/8 of 14″) potato chips, 1 oz. salad dressing—Italian, 1 T salad dressing—Russian, 1 T salad dressing—Bleu cheese, 1 T soups-most made with whole milk, 1 c. vanilla wafers, 10
11+ grams of fat	apple snack, 3 oz. (14 g.) beef fat, 1 T (20 g.) cheese danish, 1-3 oz. (25 g.) cheesecake, 1/12 cake (18 g.)

OTHER (continued)

11+ grams of fat	cherry pie, 1/6 of 9″ (18 g.)
	chicken fat, 1 T (13 g.)
	chocolate chip cookies, 4—1.7 oz. (11 g.)
	corn oil, 1 T (14 g.)
	glazed doughnut, 1 (13 g.)
	lemon meringue pie, 1/6 of 9″ (14 g.)
	mayonnaise, 1 T (11 g.)
	olive oil, 1 T (14 g.)
	peanut oil, 1 T (14 g.)
	pound cake, 1 slice (12 g.)
	pumpkin pie, 1/6 of 9″ (17 g.)
	quiche-cheese, 1 slice (20 g.)
	shortening, 1 T (13 g.)
	spaghetti sauce, 1 c. (12 g.)
	sunflower seeds, 1 oz. (14 g.)

Weight-for-Height Age Specific Gerontology

(Age-specific weight range for men and women as recommended by the Gerontology Research Center.)

Height (ft./in.)	20-29 yrs.	30-39 yrs.	40-49 yrs.	50-59 yrs.	60-69 yrs.
4 10	84-111	92-119	99-127	107-135	115-142
4 11	87-115	95-123	103-131	111-139	119-147
5 0	90-119	98-127	106-135	114-143	123-152
5 1	93-123	101-131	110-140	118-148	127-157
5 2	96-127	105-136	113-144	122-153	131-163
5 3	99-131	108-140	117-149	126-158	135-168
5 4	102-135	112-145	121-154	130-163	140-173
5 5	106-140	115-149	125-159	134-168	144-179
5 6	109-144	119-154	129-164	138-174	148-184
5 7	112-148	122-159	133-169	143-179	153-190
5 8	116-153	126-163	137-174	147-184	158-196
5 9	119-137	130-168	141-179	151-190	162-201
5 10	122-162	134-173	145-184	136-195	167-207
5 11	126-167	137-178	149-190	160-201	172-213
6 0	129-171	141-183	153-195	165-207	177-219
6 1	133-176	145-188	157-200	169-213	182-225
6 2	137-181	149-194	162-206	174-219	187-232
6 3	141-186	153-199	166-212	179-225	192-238
6 4	144-191	157-205	171-218	184-231	197-244

From "Principles of Geriatric Medicine," R. Andres et. al. Copyright 1985, McGraw-Hill Publishing Co. Used by permission.

When you set reasonable and sensible goals for yourself, look for long term results, not short-term "quick fixes." It should not be difficult to realize a six to twelve pound weight loss during this three-month period, but the difference with this weight loss is that you can expect it to be truly long-lasting. By reducing your fat intake, you are changing your eating habits, and your body is using up the stored fat for energy needs. We are including a height/weight chart from a study released by Drs. Andres, Bierman and Hazzard (see facing page). This particular chart, from advanced studies in health and fat distribution, acknowledges the body changes from ages 20-69 and changes the weight recommendations to be specific to age groups in ten-year segments, rather than only by gender and frame size.

Always remember that any chart is merely a guide for you; 3D has always encouraged participants to ask God for the weight that He wants one to attain and maintain. Stay in reality about what is a practical and possible weight within your lifestyle and circumstances.

Where Does Cholesterol Fit In?

As an ever-increasing number of people are developing heart disease, more and more Americans are becoming concerned about their cholesterol levels. How does this fit in to a low-fat diet? By reducing the amount of fat in our diet, we can help to control our cholesterol levels—an extra side benefit for those with a high cholesterol count.

There are two types of cholesterol: Dietary cholesterol and blood cholesterol. The body tries to regulate the amount of blood cholesterol that it produces with the amount of dietary cholesterol that is taken in. The body is always producing cholesterol and produces sufficient quantities for normal body functions—manufacture of hormones, bile acid and vitamin D. If you eat a high cholesterol diet your body may not be able to adjust. Surplus cholesterol can put you "at risk" for heart disease.

The terms you have heard in connection with cholesterol is your HDL and LDL count. HDL stands for High density lipoprotein and LDL stands for Low density lipoprotein. No matter how many times you hear about HDL and LDL you don't quite know what is bad and what is good cholesterol. The simplest explanation we have heard is that h means heavy, h means high and l means light and l means low. Believe it or not it is the heavy/high cholesterol you want not the light/low cholesterol! If you are aerobically fit and your liver, where all foods go, and where cholesterol is produced, is in good shape it will be able to disguise the fats that come into your body. It will wrap protein around it before it goes into your general circulation and it will just be absorbed with the protein. Cholesterol is like wax or paraffin: if it is not properly used it will be deposited in the walls of the arteries—coronary arteries and the arteries of other vital organs (arteriosclerosis). Some kinds of fat tend to raise the cholesterol level in the blood; some types can help to keep the cholesterol level low. It is important to remember that *all* types of fat have the same caloric value, *but* they do affect your blood cholesterol level differently. **Saturated fats** tend to raise the blood cholesterol level and are found in foods of animal origin (red and dark meat, dairy products, eggs and shellfish). Saturated fat usually hardens at room temperature, so that's a good way to detect it. **Unsaturated fats** do not raise blood cholesterol, and can be found in peanut oils, canola and olive oil. They are usually liquid when refrigerated. If used as substitution for saturated fat it may help reduce blood cholesterol levels. Other unsaturated fats can be found in such oils of plant origin, as safflower, soybean, sunflower, cottonseed and corn oil. These fats, too, are usually liquid when refrigerated.

All reports indicate that overall cholesterol can be controlled by a regular exercise program, eliminating saturated fat from our diet, and keeping overall fat intake below 30% of our total daily caloric intake. (There are exceptions: the genetic factor of an individual is a major determining factor.) The program that 3D is recommending in this guide enforces these principles. Just this week a member of a pilot group using the low fat plan and the resistance training exercise reported that after three months her cholesterol level had dropped from 268 to 189! So we know it works.

In the back of this guide you will find three weeks of recipes that you can rotate or repeat during the twelve weeks. We also recommend an excellent cookbook, *The Heart Smart Cookbook,* that will count the fats for you! Until you become more knowledgeable and familiar with counting fats, stick to this cookbook and the guide. It has been our experience that, at a time when we are learning new disciplines, we seem to do a lot better with a daily menu plan in front of us. Now we will go on to the exercise information.

Introduction to Exercise
Endurance Training and Resistance Training

Twenty-one years ago, at the beginning of 3D, there was a statement in the material that read: "Exercise is required for men and recommended for women." Back then it was felt that most women were getting plenty of exercise chasing after children, cleaning house and running up and down stairs!

In the early 80's, however, Ed Haver, chief exercise physiologist at a California hospital and health center, joined the 3D programs as an exercise consultant and turned our attitudes 180° around by showing us the positive benefit exercise could have for all of us. Ed reminded us to look at the life of Jesus, who went everywhere on foot, walking many times from Galilee to Jerusalem (75 miles one way). There is no question that sustained physical exertion was a natural part of His daily life. That made those of us in 3D stop and think about whether we would truly be able to "follow Him" today, if He led us up and down those hillsides and around those lakes and mountains.

Ed also addressed the whole area of stress and the wonderful help exercise is in reducing stress. In the early '80's, stress was not the buzz word it is today, but many of us still knew we were burning out under the pressures of home, family, finances and personal needs. With Ed's help we experimented with walking daily

29

early in the morning and in less than a week not only were we all feeling much better physically but there was definite difference in all of us emotionally—stress was being released, just by walking!

In this guide we will take a giant step onward from the place Ed Haver brought us in 1980—to a resistance exercise training program. So take a deep breath, open your minds, and together let's see what God has for us!

There are two main types of exercise—endurance training and resistance training. Endurance training is "aerobic" with oxygen or cardiovascular exercise. In this type, you contract large muscle groups many times against little resistance other than gravity. In order to supply enough oxygen to these working muscles your heart rate and blood pressure increases making your cardiovascular system function more efficiently. And since the most important muscle in your body is your heart, endurance exercise is vital! Walking, jogging, cycling, dancing, cross country skiing, rowing, swimming, and even stair-climbing are all examples of endurance activities.

Aerobic exercise does not require excessive speed or muscular strength. Huffing and puffing is often identified with it and that's good, because it means you are demanding your heart work harder and that demand requires something of your respiratory and circulatory systems—end result: a healthier heart! 3D participants have been committed to walking at least three times per week for at least 30 minutes, and this discipline should continue without interruption; we are adding something to your fitness program, not taking anything away.

Resistance training is anaerobic—literally "without oxygen." Resistance exercise is based on the principle that your body adapts to the amount of stress put on it, and this stress is needed to produce improvement in muscle strength, and flexibility. The muscle responds and gains strength. Without an exercise program, the muscles will shrink and weaken just by getting older. This type

30

of program will increase your range of motion and your flexibility—not to mention the highly desirable results in the fat burning department of your body.

The specific resistance training exercise that 3D will be introducing in this breakthrough program is weight lifting. You probably have never considered doing weight lifting, and the immediate image that comes up in your mind is a body builder. But lifting weights two or three times a week will not turn you into a body-builder! The great value of this type of program is that you get your muscles working—often when they haven't really worked in years. And when your muscles get activated, they burn sugar and fat together, and begin to demand more fat for energy, and guess what? The body goes into the fat storage tanks for the needed fuel.

In some of us exercise brings up all kinds of negative feelings. "I feel fat" . . . "I look awful in sweats," . . . "I feel clumsy," . . . "I feel ashamed," . . . "I feel silly." . . . So take comfort—a lot of other people entering an exercise program have the same types of feelings running around in their minds as you may. They are normal reactions; everyone feels self-conscious at first—especially when you put on a sweat suit and nothing is hidden from sight. The thighs are filling the pant leg out to the maximum—the hips are just sitting there as exposed as can be, and even if you have a half decent waist it is hidden under the sweatshirt! Emotionally most of us with weight problems have a lot to do in just accepting ourselves. If we will face the facts, then we can do something about getting those fat cells moving and converting the fat to muscle. The good news is: we do not have to talk or think dieting. We do have to think exercise.

We have had several pilot groups going with a combination of the new low fat program and a resistance-training program. And every emotion that you will have, we can guarantee has already been experienced—and expressed—in these pilot groups. Initially

31

we all looked around at each other and tried to make ourselves comfortable—while feeling so uncomfortable! We went up to the local discount store and bought our sweats and our weights and felt sure everyone in the store was wondering what these "old fat" ladies were doing with sweats and weights. Well, what is old and what is fat? It just depends on your own personal opinion. The feelings are the same, if you are 20 years old at 128 lbs comparing yourself to a 20-year old weighing only 105 lbs. or 50 years old weighing 145 comparing yourself to a 50 year old weighing 130. Facts versus feelings! Feelings can be so deceiving! I doubt there was a single person in the whole store looking at me, as I bought the sweat suit and the five-pound dumbbells.

Now for the good news: In the first pilot group with seven women, in 12 weeks there was a weight loss of 63 pounds and a total of 49 inches lost! The weights used in that first pilot program were five pound dumbbells. Simply by lowering the fat intake in daily food and doing a resistance training program two days a week in addition to continuing the walking, members of the pilot groups saw excellent results. Other pilot groups continue to bring in good results: weight loss, inches lost, more energy, better sleep, stronger arms for lifting children or groceries, and lower backs definitely strengthened where they had been weak.

One group with men and women over 55 has seen astounding results: a woman with cancer says, "I feel like I have my own body back," a man who had been using a cane is now walking totally unassisted, and a woman with a bad knee is climbing stairs— "for the first time I can go upstairs like a normal person." Those are some of the physical needs that have been met within the resistance training group, and literally everyone in the pilot programs is feeling better emotionally!

In these next 12 weeks, we want you to start working out with weights. We recommend that you purchase a set of five pound dumbbells (they cost about a dollar a pound) and follow the program in this guide, twice a week as a group. A recent *Readers' Digest* article, "The S Factor: A Dieter's Dream" (see insert article in this guide), says that strength training is a dieter's dream, because for every pound of flab that you replace with muscle, you burn dozens of extra calories per week. The reason: muscle tissue is more metabolically active—muscle cells have more chemical reactions that fat cells do. Muscle cells, even at rest, burn more energy than fat cells.

Exercising with weights is a new thing for many men and even more woman, but the benefits are many: reversal of symptoms of osteoporosis, loss of muscle tissue, arthritis, frailty, fatigue, and poor balance, just to name a few. For women who tend to be especially weak in the upper part of their bodies, weight-lifting will greatly increase the strength in their arms and back.

From warmup to cool-down, your weight exercises should last 30-45 minutes. Your aerobic activity should be 30 minutes on other days of the week. The resistance training sessions should be spaced by at least one day in order to rest your muscles.

The ideal sequence in which to exercise is to stretch first, then to do some form of aerobic exercise, and then do the weight resistance exercise. This would give you a one hour exercise class twice a week. In the pilot groups we have added a half-hour onto one of our classes to have a time of sharing. Spiritually, we continue the disciplines of prayer for each other every day, and the reading daily of our 3D devotional book. (If this is a first time class, and you have more than six members, you may also have to add a half-hour on to your second class as well, to keep the spiritual support group emphasis.) And group leaders need to check over the daily fat diaries, outside of class. With members only recording fat intake, this task is simple.

People who have been a part of 3D for years and years are entering into this new dual program with excitement, enthusiasm, and good results. If you are brand new to 3D, you have come

33

aboard at "breakthrough" time! A program with a new vision is just beginning, and you are going to be a part of it. And you can expect more to come to reinforce what we are beginning in this guide.

The following pages explain the exercises we recommend for your class.

Author's Note

Not all exercise programs are suitable for everyone, and with this or any other program, injury is possible.

Therefore, before undertaking this or any other program of exercise, you should consult your personal physician. The instructions given in this program are not intended to be a substitute for personal, professional advice.

The creators, publishers and distributors of this program disclaim any loss, liability and expense which may be incurred in connection with the exercises or instructions contained herein.

Resistance Training Exercises

Warmup

This section is designed to warm your body up. The exercises contained in this section are aimed at each part of your body and will enable you to stretch your muscles and limber up your body. The warmup and short cool-down are the two most important parts so be sure not to skip either, even though they appear simple. The warmup prevents injury to your muscles and the cool down allows your heart to slow down gradually.

Remember to breath in through the nose and out through the mouth. It is easy to just hold your breath or breathe erratically while exercising which drives your blood pressure up! We often think we should be holding our breath when we lift and breathing out when we put something down. It is the opposite—breath out when lifting and breath in when putting something down. So do concentrate on breathing correctly. Also, while doing exercises in a standing position, stand up straight and keep stomach muscles pulled in tight!

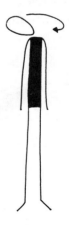

Head Rolls:
Drop your head and rotate right (right shoulder, front, left shoulder, back and then right shoulder). Repeat. Then reverse and do same movement to the left two times.

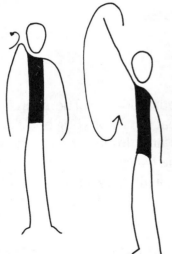

Shoulder rolls:

Lift and rotate right shoulder back followed by rotating extended right arm up and back, lift and rotate left shoulder back followed by rotating extended left arm up and back, lift and rotate both shoulders back and follow with rotating both arms extended up and back. Repeat for a total of four times.

Stretch to Heaven:

Raise both arms over head, grab your right wrist with your left hand and stretch twice, using your left hand to gently pull your right arm upward. Then switch and repeat the stretch by grabbing your left wrist with your right hand. Repeat for a total of eight.

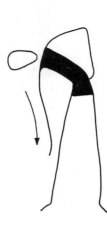

Slide Stretch:

Keep feet shoulder width apart, arms down at sides, bend to the right and slide arm down right leg, while left arm slides up. Repeat to the left. Do this exercise alternating sides for a total of eight. Remember to keep your stomach muscles pulled in tightly.

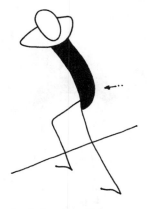

Calf stretch:

Stand arms length from something you can lean against. You can lean on it with your forearms and rest your head on your forearms if you wish. Bend one leg and put the foot on the ground by the wall, with other leg straight out behind you. Slowly move your hips forward, keeping your lower back flat. Be sure to try to keep the heel of the back leg on the ground with toes pointed straight ahead as you hold the stretch. You should feel some stretching down at the bottom back of your lower extended leg. Hold for 15 seconds. Then reverse leg positions. Hold 15 seconds.

Quad Stretch:

Grab your right foot with your right hand and bring up behind your seat and hold for a count of eight. Now, lower your right foot and grab your left foot with your left hand and bring it up behind your seat and hold for a count of eight. Repeat 2 x.

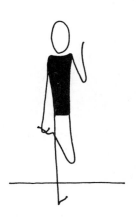

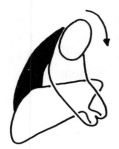

Inner thigh stretch:

Sitting on the floor legs in front, soles touching each other move your feet towards your body with soles still together until you feel slight tension in inner thigh. Then lean forward gently, hold 15 seconds to complete stretch.

37

Hamstring stretch:

Feet shoulder width apart. With your knees slightly bent with seat tucked under,(this is very important so you don't hurt your lower back) slowly bend forward from the hips. Let your neck and your arms relax as you bend forward and reach down until you feel a slight stretch in the back of your upper legs. Hold for 15 seconds...... no bouncing. Keep your knees bent as you stand up.

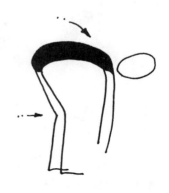

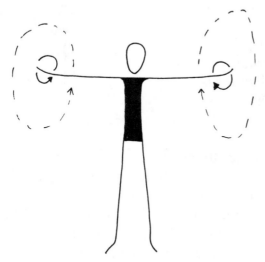

Small and Large Arm Circles:

Stand with feet shoulder width apart, extend arms shoulder height and make 8 small circles forward and 8 small circles backwards and repeat. Follow this by making 4 large circles forward and 4 large circles backwards and repeat.

Elbow extensions:

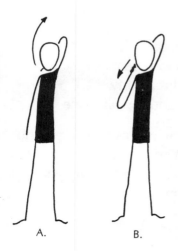

A.   B.

Standing with feet shoulder width apart, extend your right arm over your head. Bend arm at elbow down behind your head and extend back up again. Repeat for a total of 8 times. Now switch arms and extend your left arm over your head.

Bend arm at elbow down behind your head and extend back up again. Repeat for a total of 8 times. Now repeat entire exercise.

Twists:

With arms relaxed at side and knees slightly bent turn upper body gently to the left swinging arms out and swing to the right repeating arm movement. Do a total of twenty twists.

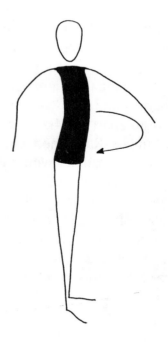

Now you are warmed up and ready to start your resistance training exercises.

39

Resistance Exercise

Week 1: Do each exercise 10 times (1 set).
Week 2-3: Do each exercise 10 times and repeat.
Week 4: Do each exercise 10 times and repeat twice.
Week 5-12: Do each exercise 12 times and repeat twice.

It is important to bring the weights down slowly. You will notice that the count of 2 is used for the first movement and the count of 4 to complete the exercise. Remember to rest before each "set" of 10 if you do each exercise more than once.

Using 5 lb. weights in each hand do the following exercises:

Side Flys: This exercise will primarily work the shoulder muscles.

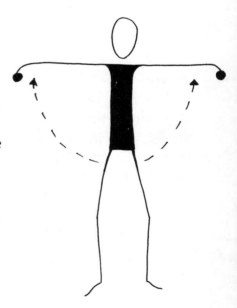

Holding the 5# weights in each hand stand with your feet shoulder width apart and hands relaxed on side of thighs. Raise the weights to the top of your shoulder with palms facing the floor, keeping both arms parallel to the floor. Return hands to starting position. Keep knees slight bent. The exercise count is up to the shoulder in 2 counts exhaling while lifting—and take 4 counts to return to starting position while inhaling.

Bicep Curl: This exercise will strengthen front of arms, and also wrists and forearms.

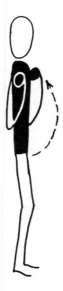

   Stand with feet shoulder width apart and knees slightly bent, holding the 5# weights with the arms relaxed at your side. Curl your forearm to your shoulders, keeping elbows stationary ending with palms facing chest. Return to starting position by lowering weights to your side. Exhale when you lift up for 2 counts and inhale as you lower for 4 counts.

Military Press: This exercise will strengthen your triceps or muscles at the back of your arms.

   Standing with feet shoulder width apart, holding 5# dumbbell in each hand at shoulder height. The elbows are bent and the palms face forward. Knees are slightly bent. Press up with the weights and extend arm overhead, never fully extending but keep arm slightly bent. Return to starting position. Exhale as you press up for 2 counts and inhale as you lower to shoulder for 4 counts.

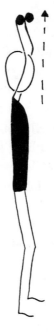

41

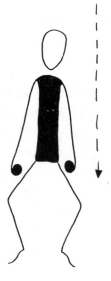

Squats: This exercise will strengthen upper thighs, buttocks and back.

Holding your 5# weights in each hand and relaxed at your side, stand with feet shoulder width apart, toes slightly turned out so knees are over feet. Knees slightly bent. Slowly lower your body by bending knees, keeping heels on floor with your shoulder back and seat tucked under. Exhale down for 2 counts and inhale up to starting position for 2 counts.

Crunches: This exercise will strengthen the abdominal muscles.

Week 1: Do 25 crunches
Week 2-3: Do 2 sets of 30 crunches each
Week 4: Do 3 sets of 35 crunches each
Week 5-12: Do 3 sets of 40 crunches each

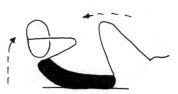

Lie on floor with back and buttocks resting on floor and pull knees towards chest feet crossed at ankles. (This helps keep lower back supported by pressing it into floor.) Arms are behind your head or crossed on your chest. Raise shoulders off floor and move towards upper legs exhaling. Inhale as you lower upper body to floor. This is really a short range movement. Do not use your neck or your arms to pull your upper body off floor, only your stomach muscles.

TIP: Always keep your stomach muscles pulled in (contracted) as you perform this exercise.

Cool Down

End with a 5-10 minute cool down. The cool down will enable you to relax and bring your heart rates down from your workout level.

Head Rolls:
Drop your head and rotate right, back, left. Repeat. Then reverse and do same movement to the left two times.

Waist Rolls:
Place hands on hips with feet shoulder width apart and bend forward at waist. Rotate body right, back, left and forward. Repeat. Then reverse and rotate body left, back, right and forward. Repeat.

Rag Doll Shake:
Hang over heavy and walk hands around behind your right heel and hold. Walk hands around behind left heel and hold. Walk hands center and pause with palms on floor, bend knees and stand.

You have completed your resistance training exercise program from warm up to cool down. As previously mentioned, you should follow this particular program twice a week, continue walking two to three times a week and follow a low fat eating plan. We know you will be blessed with a new outlook on this whole area of your life.

Appendix

Twenty-One Days of Simple, Easy-to-Plan, Low Fat Meals

DAY 1

Breakfast: 1/2 grapefruit
1 oz rice or oat cereal with skim milk
1/2 cup nonfat yogurt

Lunch: French Market Soup (recipe on pg 55 in guide)
Roll

Dinner: Tomato juice
Stir fry chicken with snow peas
1/2 c rice
wedge of lettuce with low fat dressing

DAY 2

Breakfast: 2 slices whole wheat toast with sugar free jam
1 orange
1/2 c no fat cottage cheese

Lunch: Chefs salad with 2 oz cheese
Non-fat salad dressing
3 crackers

45

Dinner: Whitefish with Wine and Peppercorns (pg 183 Heart
               Smart)
            Green beans
            Large Baked potato with no fat sour cream or Molly
               McButter

DAY 3

Breakfast: Bagel with no fat cream cheese
            sliced banana with skim milk

Lunch: Ambrosia Fruit Salad (pg 104 Heart Smart)
            hard roll (no more than 4 grams of fat)

Dinner: Turkey Lasagna (pg 201 Heart Smart)
            Tossed Salad with low fat dressing

DAY 4

Breakfast: 1/3 cantaloupe
            1 oz cereal with skim milk

Lunch: English muffin
            2 oz tuna packed in water
            mixed with no fat mayo
            Melt no fat cheese on top if desired
            Sliced pineapple

Dinner: Stuffed baked potato with cheese and broccoli
            Applesauce
            Celery/carrot sticks

DAY 5

Breakfast: 2 slices french toast made with egg beaters
            3/4 cup fresh strawberries

Lunch: Gazpacho (pg 86 Heart Smart)
            Roll or crackers

Dinner: Beef and Macaroni Casserole (pg 155 Heart Smart)
           Fresh Asparagus

DAY 6

Breakfast: 3/4 c oatmeal with skim milk
           raisins
           Orange juice

Lunch: Herbed Chicken Salad (pg 100 Heart Smart)
           Green grapes and 1/6 cantaloupe
           Roll

Dinner: Spinach Calzones (pg 131 Heart Smart)
           Sliced tomatoes and lettuce with low fat dressing

DAY 7

Breakfast: 2 EGGO waffles
           1/2 c no-fat cottage cheese

Lunch: Shrimp and Rice Salad (recipe on page 59 in guide)
           Sliced orange

Dinner: Meatloaf
           Baked Potato
           Sliced carrots/Peas

DAY 8

Breakfast: 1 poached egg on toast
           1/2 grapefruit

Lunch: Pita bread with leftover vegetables and no fat cheese
           melted

Dinner: 6 Ounces broiled fish
           pasta (angel hair or noodles)
           1 cup steamed spinach

DAY 9

Breakfast: Breakfast Casserole (recipe on pg 58 in guide)

Lunch: Hearty Chicken Vegetable Soup (can)
4 saltine crackers
Apple

Dinner: Chicken Dijon (recipe on pg 54 in guide)
Rice
Broccoli

DAY 10

Breakfast: 3/4 c cold cereal with skim milk
1 piece of toast with jam
1/2 banana

Lunch: Pasta with low fat spaghetti sauce
Tossed Salad with low fat dressing

Dinner: Marinated Scallop Kabobs (pg 185 Heart Smart)
Rice

DAY 11

Breakfast: Shredded wheat cereal with skim milk
Strawberries

Lunch: Reuben sandwich:
1 oz canned corned beef
1/4 cup drained sauerkraut
1 oz low fat Swiss cheese
1 oz no fat Russian dressing

Dinner: Fettucini Parmesan with Vegetable (pg 193 Heart Smart)
Italian bread
Squash

DAY 12

Breakfast: Bagel with no fat cream cheese
1/2 grapefruit

Lunch: 1 cup clam chowder (canned)
crackers or roll
Pear

Dinner: Roast Turkey (slice and freeze in 3 ounce portions for lunches, etc.)
Sweet Potato
Brussels sprouts
Cranberry sauce

DAY 13

Breakfast: 3/4 cup oatmeal with skim milk
1/3 cantaloupe or honeydew

Lunch: Large wheat tortilla with deli turkey, lettuce, tomato
Microwave Potato Chips (recipe on page 62 in guide)

Dinner: Chicken Hot Dog in roll
3/4 cup baked beans

DAY 14

Breakfast: Blueberry-Yogurt Muffin (recipe on page 54 in guide)
1 boiled egg
Orange juice

Lunch: Greek salad with low fat dressing
Pita bread

Dinner: Stirfry chicken with broccoli and carrots
Rice pilaf
Mandarin oranges with pineapple chunks

DAY 15

Breakfast: Cold cereal of your choice with skim milk and 1/2 banana
Pineapple juice

Lunch: Grilled cheese (low fat cheese)
Sliced tomatoes with lettuce wedges, cucumbers

Dinner: Barbecue Chicken (pg 137 Heart Smart)
Noodles
Broccoli with cauliflower and carrots

DAY 16

Breakfast: Entenmann's coffee cake 1/2" slice
1/3 cantaloupe with no fat cottage cheese

Lunch: Sliced turkey sandwich with cranberry sauce

Dinner: Pasta Primavera (recipe on page 63 in guide)
Green beans with mushrooms

DAY 17

Breakfast: 1 Apple Muffin (recipe on pg 64 in guide)
1/2 c cottage cheese

Lunch: Sliced cantaloupe and honeydew and strawberries
1 cup yogurt
Hard roll

Dinner: Corn chowder made with turkey (recipe on pg. 62 in guide)
Corn bread

DAY 18

Breakfast: French toast made with egg beaters
Sliced peaches

Lunch: Ambrosia Fruit Salad (pg 104 Heart Smart)
Bed of lettuce
Choice of crackers

Dinner: Turkey Chili (pg 151 Heart Smart)
            Corn bread with honey

DAY 19

Breakfast: 1/2 cantaloupe with cottage cheese and pineapple chunks
            1/2 English muffin with jam

Lunch: Tuna Salad sandwich
            Sliced tomato with lettuce with low fat dressing

Dinner: Pizza with Sauce Classico (pg 129 Heart Smart)
            Tossed salad with low fat dressing (any fresh vegetables
                available)

DAY 20

Breakfast: Cream of wheat cereal with skim milk
            Orange juice

Lunch: Healthy choice vegetable soup
            Crackers
            Apple

Dinner: Layered Cabbage/Beef Casserole (pg 168 Heart Smart)
            Roll
            Green Beans

DAY 21

Breakfast: 1 poached egg on toast
            Cranberry juice

Lunch: Deli turkey sandwich on onion roll
            Sliced tomato
            Lettuce

Dinner: Stuffed peppers with either ground turkey or Healthy
                choice hamburg
            Peas
            Salad with low fat dressing

The *Heart Smart Cookbook* is filled with wonderful recipes and substitutions are encouraged.

Herbs and Seasonings will be a tremendous help in cooking the low fat way. Fresh herbs are always wonderful but dried herbs will serve most purposes of enhancing the dish to be served. Wine used for poaching adds flavor with no calories. Also, use no fat spray for stir frying of meats or vegetables.

Low Fat Desert Choices
Festive Fruitcake (recipe on page 60 in guide)
All fresh fruits (no limit)
No Guilt Brownies (recipe on pg 55 in guide)
Frozen yogurt
Baked apples
Angel food cake
Cakes made with applesauce or crushed pineapple as substitute ingredients for oil
Puddings made with skim milk
Entenmann's no fat pound cake/oatmeal raisin cookies

Recipes

Egg Beaters Cheese Soufflé

¼ c butter or margarine (reduce to 3 T)
¼ c flour, scant
½ t salt
dash cayenne
1 c milk (may need a bit more)
8 oz Fat Free Cheese (about 10 slices)
1 box (8 oz) Egg Beaters
2 egg whites

Melt butter; blend in flour, salt and cayenne. Add milk all at once. Cook over medium heat, stirring until thick and bubbly. Remove from heat, Add cheese; stir until cheese melts (if too stiff add a bit more milk). Beat Egg Beaters. Slowly add cheese mixture, stirring constantly. Beat eggs to stiff peaks. Gradually pour eggbeater mixture over; fold together well. Pour into ungreased soufflé dish or casserole (2 qt.) Bake at 300° 1-1¼ hr. until knife inserted off-center comes out clean. Break apart into servings with 2 forks.

Yield: 4-6   3.4 grams fat per serving

Curried Lima Beans

2 pkg frozen baby lima beans
1 c water
2 T unsalted butter
1 medium onion, chopped (½ c)
4 t curry powder
¼ c plain yogurt
4 t lemon juice
¼ t salt
¼ t black pepper

Bring water and beans to boil in medium saucepan over high heat. Lower heat, cover and cook for 6 minutes. Drain beans, set aside. Melt butter in same saucepan over medium heat. Add onion and curry powder; cook, stirring occasionally, 6-8 minutes or until onion is tender. Stir in limas until heated through. Remove from heat. Stir in yogurt, lemon juice, salt and pepper until well combined and heated through. Serve immediately.

Yield: 4-6   3 grams fat per serving

Blueberry-Yogurt Muffins

2 c all-purpose flour
$^1/_3$ c sugar
1 t baking powder
1 t baking soda
¼ t salt
¼ c unsweetened orange juice
2 T vegetable oil
1 t vanilla extract
1 (8-oz) carton vanilla low-fat yogurt
1 egg
1 c fresh or frozen blueberries
Vegetable cooking spray
1 T sugar

Combine the first 5 ingredients in a large bowl; make a well in center of mixture.
Combine orange juice and next 4 ingredients; stir well. Add to dry ingredients, stirring just until moistened. Gently fold in blueberries. Divide batter evenly among 12 muffin cups coated with cooking spray; sprinkle 1 T sugar evenly over muffins. Bake at 400° for 18 minutes or until golden. Remove from pans immediately; let cool on a wire rack.

Yield: 1 dozen   3 grams fat per muffin

Chicken Dijon

6 chicken breasts split
3 T flour
1½-2 c chicken broth
¾ c non-fat sour cream
4 T Dijon mustard
2 tomatoes cut in wedges
2 T minced parsley

Brown chicken on both sides in broiler until well cooked. Remove to a platter and then make sauce with drippings, flour, sour cream and chicken broth to desired thickness. Put chicken back in pan and cook in 325° oven until all cooked and hot. Decorate with tomatoes and parsley to serve.

Yield: 12   8 grams fat each

French Market Soup

1 (12 oz) pkg dried bean soup
9 c water
1 c cubed lean cooked ham
½ t salt
¼ t white pepper
1 (16 oz) whole tomatoes
1½ c chopped onion
¾ c chopped celery
2 large cloves garlic, minced
3 T lemon juice
1 t hot sauce

Sort and wash bean soup mix; place in Dutch oven. cover with water 2 inches above beans; let soak 8 hours.
Drain beans and return to Dutch oven. Add 9 c water, ham, salt and white pepper.
Bring to a boil; reduce heat and simmer, uncovered, 2 hours or until beans are tender.
Chop tomatoes and add with remaining ingredients; simmer 30 minutes, stirring occasionally.

Yield: 6 servings (1½ c each).   2.9 grams fat per 1½ cups

No Guilt Brownies

3 oz unsweetened chocolate, chopped
1 c granulated sugar
¾ c flour
¾ c fat-free cottage cheese
3 egg whites
1 t salt
powdered sugar

Heat oven to 350°. Over very low heat, melt chocolate; cool slightly. In food processor, purée all ingredients except chocolate and powdered sugar until smooth. Add melted chocolate. Blend well. Pour into lightly buttered 8″ square pan. Bake 20-25 minutes or until just set. Sprinkle with powdered sugar. Cut into 16 squares.

1 gram fat per square

55

Cornmeal Yeast Muffins

1 pkg dry yeast
¼ c warm water (105-115°)
1¹/₃ c skim milk
¹/₃ c sugar
¼ c vegetable oil
¼ c margarine
1 t salt
½ c egg substitute
1½ c plain cornmeal
5-5½ c all-purpose flour, divided
Vegetable spray

Dissolve yeast in warm water in large bowl; let stand 5 minutes. Combine milk and next 4 ingredients in saucepan; cook over low heat until margarine melts. Cool to 105-115°. Add milk mixture to yeast mixture. Stir in egg substitute, corn meal, 2 c flour. Beat at medium speed with electric mixer until smooth. Stir in enough remaining flour to make a soft dough. Turn dough out onto a lightly floured surface and knead until smooth and elastic (about 8 min.). Place in a bowl coated with cooking spray, turning to grease top. Cover and let rise in warm place (85°), free from drafts, 1 hour or until doubled in bulk. Punch down dough; shape in 72 balls. Place 2 balls in muffin cup coated with spray. Let rise in warm place (85°), free from drafts, 45 min. or until doubled in bulk. Bake at 375° for 12-15 minutes or until golden. Coat muffins with cooking spray, remove from pans immediately. Serve or freeze.

Yield: 3 dozen   2.8 grams fat per muffin

Baked Apple

Large fresh apple
brown sugar
raisins (as desired)
sugar & cinnamon

Core apple, place in bowl. Sprinkle with cinnamon & sugar. Spoon brown sugar and raisins in opening. Microwave 3-4 minutes. May top with non-fat yogurt.

0 grams fat

Shrimp Stir-Fry with Ginger-Orange Sauce

1¼ lb medium-sized fresh unpeeled shrimp
vegetable cooking spray
4 c sliced yellow squash
1 c sliced zucchini
²/₃ c chopped red bell pepper
½ c diagonally sliced celery
½ lb pre-sliced fresh mushrooms
2 T cornstarch
1 T brown sugar
3 T reduced-sodium soy sauce
1 (10½ oz) can low-sodium chicken broth
2 cloves garlic, minced
2-3 t grated fresh gingerroot or ⅛ to ½ t ground ginger
6 c hot cooked rice (cooked without salt or fat)

Peel and devein shrimp. Coat a large non-stick skillet with cooking spray, and place over medium-high heat until hot. Add shrimp; stir-fry 2 minutes. Remove from skillet and set aside. Combine yellow squash, zucchini, bell pepper, celery and mushrooms; add half of vegetables to skillet. Stir-fry 3 min. over medium-high heat. Remove from skillet, and set aside. Repeat procedure with remaining vegetables; stir-fry 3 minutes and set aside. Combine cornstarch, brown sugar, soy sauce and chicken broth; stir well. Add garlic and ginger to skillet; sauté 30 seconds. Add cornstarch mixture; bring to a boil, stirring constantly. Cook 1 minute or until thickened. Stir in shrimp and vegetables; cook 1 minute. Serve over rice.

Yield: 6 servings (1 c shrimp mixture/1 c rice)   2.4 grams fat per serving

Turkey Tortilla

1 wheat tortilla
1 slice deli turkey
mustard or dijonaise
lettuce
sliced tomato

Spread mustard or dijonaise on tortilla. Add turkey and other ingredients as desired. Roll-up!

3 minute preparation   Yield: 1   1 gram fat

Breakfast Casserole

3 c cubed French bread
vegetable cooking spray
¾ c diced lean cooked ham
1 c (4 oz.) shredded, reduced fat sharp cheddar cheese
1¹/₃ c skim milk
¾ c egg substitute
¼ t dry mustard
¼ t onion powder
¼ t white pepper
paprika

Place bread evenly in 8" square baking dish coated with cooking spray. Layer ham, red pepper and cheese over bread. Set aside. Combine next 4 ingredients; pour over cheese. Cover and refrigerate 8 hours. Remove from refrigerator; let stand 30 minutes. Bake, uncovered, at 350° for 30 minutes; sprinkle with paprika. Serve immediately.

Yield: 6 ¾-c servings   5 grams fat per serving

Meat Loaf

²/₃ c dry bread crumbs
1 c skim milk
1½ lbs ground turkey
½ c egg substitute
¼ t onion
1 t salt
½ t sage
pepper
Sauce
3 T brown sugar
¼ c catsup
¼ t nutmeg
1 t dry mustard

Mix all ingredients (except sauce) together well; mix sauce ingredients together. Pour sauce over meatloaf. Place in 350° oven for 45 minutes.

Yield: 4 servings   13 grams fat per serving

Shrimp and Rice Salad

3 c water
1 lb unpeeled, medium-size fresh shrimp
2 c cooked white rice
½ c chopped celery
½ c chopped green pepper
¼ c sliced pimento stuffed olives
¼ c chopped onion
2 T diced pimento
3 T oil-free Italian dressing
2 T reduced calorie or fat free mayonnaise
2 T prepared mustard
1 T lemon juice
1 t lemon-pepper seasoning
⅛ t pepper
Lettuce leaves

Bring water to boil; add shrimp and cook 3-5 minutes or until shrimp turns pink. Drain well; rinse with cold water. Chill. Peel and devein shrimp. Combine shrimp and next 6 ingredients in a medium bowl. Combine Italian dressing and next 5 ingredients, stirring until well blended. Pour over shrimp mixture, and toss gently to coat. Cover and chill 3-4 hours. Line a serving plate with lettuce leaves. Spoon salad onto plate.

Yield: 5 1-c servings   3.1 grams fat per serving

3 oz. Chicken Breasts

Season with herbs as desired. Pour ⅓ c chablis over in pan. Simmer 3-4 minutes, turning once. Serve with rice, pasta or baked potato.

4-6 grams fat

59

Festive Fruitcake

¼ c brandy
1 (6 oz) can frozen unsweetened orange juice concentrate,
    thawed and undiluted
1 c fresh cranberries, chopped
1 (8 oz) package pitted dates, chopped
1 c chopped pecans
1 T grated orange rind
1 t vanilla extract
½ c egg substitute
1 (8 oz) can unsweetened pineapple tidbits, drained
2 c all-purpose flour
1¼ t baking soda
¼ t salt
½ t cinnamon
¼ t nutmeg
¼ t allspice
vegetable cooking spray
½ c brandy
3 T apple brandy

Combine first 3 ingredients in large bowl; cover and let stand 1 hour. Combine dates and next 5 ingredients; stir into cranberry mixture. Combine flour and next 5 ingredients. Stir into fruit mixture. Spoon batter into a 6-cup Bundt or tube pan coated with cooking spray; bake at 325° for 45 minutes or until wooden pick inserted in center of cake comes out clean. Cool in pan on wire rack 20 minutes; remove from pan and let cool completely on wire rack. Bring ½ c brandy to boil; cool. Moisten several layers of cheese cloth with brandy and wrap cake. Cover with plastic wrap, then aluminum foil. Store in a cool place at least 1 week, or freeze up to 3 months. Before serving, melt apple jelly in a saucepan over low heat, stirring constantly. Brush over cake.

Yield: 21 servings   4.1 grams fat per serving

Tortillas

2 flour tortillas
4 T saucepan beans
Salsa of choice
non-fat sour cream
2 slices non-fat cheese

Put 2 T of beans and a generous portion of salsa in each tortilla and roll. Lay 1 slice of cheese on each tortilla. Add more salsa or microwave about 1.5 minutes. Add dollup of sour cream. Enjoy with a handful (approx. 26) of guiltless tortilla chips.

Yield: 2 servings   4.5 grams fat per serving

Mexican Rice and Beans

1 t canola oil
½ c water
1 onion chopped
2 cloves garlic, minced
1½ c mushrooms, sliced
2 sweet peppers, chopped
¾ c long-grain rice
1 can (28 oz) red kidney beans, drained
1 can (19 oz) tomatoes
1 T chili powder
2 t cumin
¼ t cayenne pepper
1 c shredded low-fat mozzarella cheese
Optional
1 small can whole kernel corn
¼ c red wine

In large skillet or Dutch oven, heat oil with water over medium heat. Add onion, garlic, mushrooms and green peppers; simmer, stirring often, until onion is tender, about 10 minutes. Add rice, beans, tomatoes, chili powder, cumin and cayenne (also optional items). Simmer 25 minutes or until rice is tender and most of the liquid is absorbed. Transfer to baking dish and sprinkle with cheese. Bake in 350° oven for 15 minutes or micowave on high for 1-2 minutes or until cheese melts.

Yield: 6 1-c servings.   5 grams fat per serving

61

Corn Chowder

2 T margarine
1 c chicken boullion
2 medium onions
2 cloves garlic, chopped
½ c celery, chopped
1 pepper, chopped, seeds & membranes removed
1 lb ground turkey
1½ t cayenne pepper
1½ t fennel seed, crushed
1 t coarse ground pepper
6 medium potatoes, raw, pared & diced
4 c chicken boullion or stock
½ t salt
½ t paprika
2 bay leaves
3 c skim milk
3 16-oz cans of whole kernel corn, drained
1 c instant potato buds

In margarine and boullion, sauté onions, garlic, celery and pepper. Add ground turkey, cayenne pepper, fennel seed and pepper. Sauté until brown and any liquid is gone. Add potatoes, boullion, salt, paprika and bay leaves. In separate saucepan, combine until blended skim milk and corn and bring to the boiling point. When potatoes are tender (about 45 minutes), add this milk mixture to base. Reheat, but do not boil. Slowly add potato buds (1 c more or less) until desired consistency is achieved. Stir until smooth.

Yield: 12-14 servings.   Approx. 4 grams fat per serving

Microwave Potato Chips

Unpeeled potatoes

Slice potatoes very thinly. Use 9 X 13 pyrex pan upside down. Spray with Pam. Cover with potato slices and sprinkle with salt. Cook on high for 4-7 minutes until light brown. Cool one minute.

0 grams fat

Pasta Primavera

3 c broccoli florets, cut into bite-sized pieces
½ lb fresh mushrooms, quartered
2 small zucchini, sliced into ¼" rounds
1 T olive oil
3 cloves garlic, minced
1 pt cherry tomatoes, stemmed and cut in half
8 oz fettucine

Sauce

¾ c skim milk
3 T nonfat "butter" granules (i.e. Molly McButter)
²/₃ c part-skim ricotta cheese
¼ c grated Parmesan cheese
2 T chopped fresh basil *or* 1 T dried basil
¼ c dry sherry

Steam broccoli, mushrooms and zucchini for 3 minutes or until just tender. Set aside. In large nonstick skillet or wok, heat olive oil over medium-high heat. Add garlic and sauté for 1 minute, stirring frequently. Add tomatoes and sauté for 2 minutes, stirring frequently until tomatoes are slightly cooked, but not wilted. Set aside. Cook fettucine according to package directions, omitting salt. Drain well. Combine milk, "butter" granules, ricotta cheese, parmesan cheese, basil and sherry in blender. Process until smooth. In small saucepan, heat sauce over low heat, stirring frequently, until warm. In large serving dish, toss drained pasta, vegetables and sauce to coat well. Garnish each portion with Parmesan cheese and pepper. Serve immediately.

Yield: 4 2-cup servings.   2 grams fat per serving

Apple Muffins

2 c all-purpose flour
¼ c plus 2 T firmly packed brown sugar
1 t baking powder
½ t baking soda
½ t ground cinnamon
¼ t salt
1½ c peeled, shredded Rome apples
¹/₃ c plus 2 T nonfat buttermilk
2 T vegetable oil
1 t vanilla extract
1 egg
Vegetable cooking spray

Combine first 6 ingredients in large bowl; make well in center of mixture. Combine apple and next 4 ingredients; stir well. Add to dry ingredients, stirring until just moistened. Divide batter evenly among 12 muffin cups coated with cooking spray. Bake at 400° for 28 minutes or until a wooden pick inserted in center comes out clean. Remove from pans immediately; let cool on wire rack.

Yield: 1 dozen (Serving size 1 muffin)   3.2 grams fat

Get started on the greatest adventure of your life with the

3D Action Kit

Twelve challenging weeks of spiritual growth, healthy eating and exercise!

This kit includes:

* **Workbook** - Discover this treasure. Inspiring devotionals that touch you where you live.

* **Member's Manual** - Here's how! 112 pages of "exchange" diet plans, recipes and exercise principles.

* **3D** - Smile, God has the answer! Carol Showalter candidly tells her story; she includes her guilt, sense of failure and need. Laugh, cry and be encouraged!

* **Introduction to 3D** - Get off to a great start with this informative and upbeat tape that offers helpful hints and tips.

3D Action Kit: A New Beginning - Workbook I, 3D by Carol Showalter, Members Manual, Introduction to 3D - Audio tape   **$23.95**

Commit Yourself to a New Start

3D introduces
Action Kit II
36 weeks of life-changing devotionals

Heart of the Matter
Pressing On
Along the King's Highway

For the first time, 3D is offering **Action Kit II** to encourage you to continue in the 3D program. On its own, Action Kit II is an inspirational set for anyone looking for practical answers to real-life problems. Whether you are in a 3D group or not, these devotionals will spur you on in the Christian life. **$32.95**

Action Kit II Teaching Tapes are now available to supplement the devotionals. These six cassettes can offer additional short teachings for each week. Excellent for further personal meditation or group discussion. **$33.95**

FREE SHIPPING WITH THIS COUPON

ORDER TODAY!

Send this coupon to:
3D, P.O. Box 897, Orleans, MA 02653

or call the 3D office at:
1-800-451-5006 and be sure to mention this free shipping offer!

3D Action Kit II

Please send me _____ copies of the 3D Action Kit II at $32.95.
Please send me _____ sets of the 3D Action Kit II Teaching Tapes at $33.95.

☐ Check   ☐ Charge

Acct # _____ Exp. _____

Name _____

Address_____

City/State/Zip _____

Phone # _____

Amazing Food Secrets Revealed!

4001 Food Facts will become the most frequently used book in and out of your kitchen. *This is not a cookbook.* It's 282 pages packed with thousands of food and beverage facts, vitamin and mineral facts, supermarket facts and so much more. Perfect for shower and birthday gifts, this one book will help you with . . .

- How to skim the fat off of homemade chicken soup

- How to fix the clams that your family has dug on the beaches of Cape Cod

- How many grams of fat in a Burger King chicken sandwich

Every house needs a copy!
You won't be able to put it down!

Now you can count calories, fats and exchanges

with the

Heart Smart Cookbook

A simple approach to healthy eating from the Henry Ford Heart and Vascular Institute

Every recipe in this outstanding cookbook not only tastes excellent but provides an individual within the 3D program complete nutritional information, including food exchanges *and* fats.

To maintain good health and weight management, low fat food intake is a priority. The **Heart Smart Cookbook** is easy to refer to and will help you to incorporate low fat eating into your home and family life.

Heart Smart Cookbook **$14.95**

FREE SHIPPING WITH THIS COUPON

ORDER TODAY!

Send this coupon to:
3D, P.O. Box 897, Orleans, MA 02653

or call the 3D office at:
1-800-451-5006 and be sure to mention this free shipping offer!

Heart Smart Cookbook

Please send me _____ copies of the Heart Smart Cookbook at $14.95.

☐ Check   ☐ Charge

Acct # _____ Exp. _____

Name _____

Address_____

City/State/Zip _____

Phone # _____

3D *Diary Sheet*   Name _____   Group _____   Daily Fats _____   Week Beginning: _____

	MONDAY	TUESDAY	WEDNESDAY	THURSDAY	FRIDAY	SATURDAY	SUNDAY
BREAKFAST							
SNACK							
LUNCH							
SNACK							
DINNER							
TOTAL FATS							

3D *Diary Sheet*   Name _____   Group _____   Daily Fats _____   Week Beginning: _____

	MONDAY	TUESDAY	WEDNESDAY	THURSDAY	FRIDAY	SATURDAY	SUNDAY
BREAKFAST							
SNACK							
LUNCH							
SNACK							
DINNER							
TOTAL FATS							

3D *Diary Sheet* Name _____ Group _____ Daily Fats _____ Week Beginning: _____

	MONDAY	TUESDAY	WEDNESDAY	THURSDAY	FRIDAY	SATURDAY	SUNDAY
BREAKFAST							
SNACK							
LUNCH							
SNACK							
DINNER							
TOTAL FATS							

3D *Diary Sheet* Name _____ Group _____ Daily Fats _____ Week Beginning: _____

	MONDAY	TUESDAY	WEDNESDAY	THURSDAY	FRIDAY	SATURDAY	SUNDAY
BREAKFAST							
SNACK							
LUNCH							
SNACK							
DINNER							
TOTAL FATS							

3D *Diary Sheet* Name _____ Group _____ Daily Fats _____ Week Beginning: _____

	MONDAY	TUESDAY	WEDNESDAY	THURSDAY	FRIDAY	SATURDAY	SUNDAY
BREAKFAST							
SNACK							
LUNCH							
SNACK							
DINNER							
TOTAL FATS							

3D *Diary Sheet*   Name _____   Group _____   Daily Fats _____   Week Beginning: _____

	MONDAY	TUESDAY	WEDNESDAY	THURSDAY	FRIDAY	SATURDAY	SUNDAY
BREAKFAST							
SNACK							
LUNCH							
SNACK							
DINNER							
TOTAL FATS							

3D *Diary Sheet* Name _____ Group _____ Daily Fats _____ Week Beginning: _____

	MONDAY	TUESDAY	WEDNESDAY	THURSDAY	FRIDAY	SATURDAY	SUNDAY
BREAKFAST							
SNACK							
LUNCH							
SNACK							
DINNER							
TOTAL FATS							

3D *Diary Sheet*   Name _____   Group _____   Daily Fats _____   Week Beginning: _____

	MONDAY	TUESDAY	WEDNESDAY	THURSDAY	FRIDAY	SATURDAY	SUNDAY
BREAKFAST							
SNACK							
LUNCH							
SNACK							
DINNER							
TOTAL FATS							

3D *Diary Sheet* Name _____ Group _____ Daily Fats _____ Week Beginning: _____

	MONDAY	TUESDAY	WEDNESDAY	THURSDAY	FRIDAY	SATURDAY	SUNDAY
BREAKFAST							
SNACK							
LUNCH							
SNACK							
DINNER							
TOTAL FATS							

3D *Diary Sheet* Name _____ Group _____ Daily Fats _____ Week Beginning: _____

	MONDAY	TUESDAY	WEDNESDAY	THURSDAY	FRIDAY	SATURDAY	SUNDAY
BREAKFAST							
SNACK							
LUNCH							
SNACK							
DINNER							
TOTAL FATS							

3D *Diary Sheet* Name_____ Group_____ Daily Fats_____ Week Beginning:_____

	MONDAY	TUESDAY	WEDNESDAY	THURSDAY	FRIDAY	SATURDAY	SUNDAY
BREAKFAST							
SNACK							
LUNCH							
SNACK							
DINNER							
TOTAL FATS							

3D *Diary Sheet* Name _____ Group _____ Daily Fats _____ Week Beginning: _____

	MONDAY	TUESDAY	WEDNESDAY	THURSDAY	FRIDAY	SATURDAY	SUNDAY
BREAKFAST							
SNACK							
LUNCH							
SNACK							
DINNER							
TOTAL FATS							